Fracture Classifications in Clinical Practice

Fracture Classifications in Clinical Practice

Seyed Behrooz Mostofi

With 70 Figures

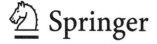 Springer

Seyed Behrooz Mostofi, FRCS (Tr & Orth)
Senior Registrar in Orthopaedics
South East Thames Rotation
University of London
United Kingdom

British Library Cataloguing in Publicaion Data
Mostofi, Seyed Behrooz
    Fracture classifications in clinical practice
    1. Fractures – Classification
    I. Title
    617.1′5′012
ISBN-10: 1846280257

Library of Congress Control Number: 2005925986

ISBN-10: 1-84628-025-7   e-ISBN: 1-84628-144-X   Printed on acid-free paper
ISBN-13: 978-1-84628-025-2

Printed in the United States of America. (BS/MVY)

9 8 7 6 5 4 3 2 1

Springer Science+Business Media
springeronline.com

This book is dedicated in loving memory of my grandparents:

Mr. Seyed Abbas Mostofi, philosopher, poet, writer and diplomat, who devoted his life to the education, happiness and well-being of others
and
Mrs. Khadijeh Mostofi, a lady of influential status, far in advance of her time, who insisted that strong moral values and a high standard of spiritual belief be maintained in her family.

God bless them.

Foreword

This is one of those necessary books to which one rushes to confirm that one's memory of fracture classification is correct. It is succinctly written and well referenced, providing a quick and easy aide memoir of fracture patterns. Drawn from many sources, a number of classifications are usefully provided for each fracture area.

Whether as a useful introduction to trauma, or as an essential prior to examination, with this book Behrooz Mostofi has produced a little gem.

Barry Hinves
Chair, Specialist Training Committee
South East Thames Rotation
University of London
United Kingdom

Preface

The staff in accident and emergency departments and doctors in fracture clinics alike may at times find themselves inadequately equipped to identify the exact type of a given fracture without access to a textbook.

Classification is an essential aid, which guides clinical judgement. It has been developed to facilitate organisation of seemingly distinct but related fractures into different clinically useful groups. Ideally, it provides a reliable language of communication guidelines for treatment, and allows reasonable progress to be drawn for a specific type of fracture. However, the "ideal" classification system that would fulfill these requirements does not exist. As a result, numerous classification systems are published for each fracture; some are more used in one geographical location than others.

This book makes no attempt to produce a comprehensive list of all classifications. Rather, it includes those practical systems which have proven helpful in everyday clinical practice to a majority of surgeons. This book aims to provide enough essential information to complete the major task of identification and analysis of fracture, which is the first step in treatment.

As other systems of classification evolve over time, the likelihood that the classifications in this book will continue to provide guidance for fracture care remains high. I accept responsibility for any shortcomings in this book and corrections will be gladly made in the next edition.

Seyed Behrooz Mostofi
London
August 2005

Acknowledgments

I am grateful to Dr. Andrée Bates whose unfailing support is a source of inspiration.

I acknowledge the help and advice of my old friend, and talented Orthopaedic Surgeon, Mr. H. Khairandish (Payman) from whom I have benefited enormously.

I am indebted to Mr. Ravi Singh, Senior Registrar in Orthopaedics for his encouragement and suggestions at the times most needed.

I am grateful to the copyright holders for their kind permission to reproduce some of the original drawings.

I would like to give special thanks to Grant Weston, Hannah Wilson, Barbara Chernow, and other staff at Springer for their support and enthusiasm for the production of this book.

Most of the uninterrupted work was done at night well into the early hours of the morning after clinics and surgery and over the weekends. Therefore, I am also appreciative of my parents, my family, especially my brother Dr. Seyed Behzad Mostofi, and friends who understood the value of this to me and forgave me for being constantly absent from social gatherings. They adjusted themselves to my difficult hours of solitary work. I am grateful to them all.

Contents

Chapter 1
Spine

CERVICAL SPINE

Injuries to the Occiput-C1–C2 Complex

Anderson and Montisano Classification of Occipital Condyle Fractures
Type I: impaction of condyle
Type II: associated with basilar or skull fractures
Type III: condylar avulsion

Atlanto-Occipital Dislocation (Craniovertebral Dissociation)

Classification Based on Position of the Occiput in Relation to C1
Type I: Occipital condyles anterior to the atlas; most common
Type II: Condyles longitudinally result of pure distraction
Type III: Occipital condyles posterior to the atlas

Atlas Fractures

Levine and Edwards Classification
1. Burst Fracture (Jefferson Fracture). Axial load injury resulting in four fractures: two in the posterior arch and two in the anterior arch.
2. Posterior arch fractures. Hyperextension injury that is associated with odontoid and axis fractures.
3. Comminuted fractures. Axial load and lateral bending injury associated with high nonunion rate and poor clinical result.
4. Anterior arch fractures. Hyperextension injury.
5. Lateral mass fractures. Axial Load and lateral bending injury.
6. Transverse process fracture. Avulsion injury.
7. Inferior tubercle fracture. Avulsion of the longus colli muscle.

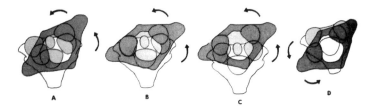

FIGURE 1.1. Fielding classification of atlantoaxial rotatory subluxation and dislocation. (Reproduced with permission and copyright © of the Journal of Bone and Joint Surgery, Inc. Fielding WJ, Hawkins RJ; Atlanto-axial rotatory fixation (Fixed rotatory subluxation of the atlanto-axial joint). *J Bone Joint Surg* 1977;59-A:37–44.)

Atlantoaxial Rotatory Subluxation and Dislocation

Fielding Classification (Figure 1.1)
Type I: Simple rotatory displacement without anterior shift. Odontoid acts as a pivot point; transverse ligament intact.
Type II: Rotatory displacement with anterior displacement of 3.5 mm. Opposite facet acts as a pivot; transverse ligament insufficient.
Type III: Rotatory displacement with anterior displacement of more than 5 mm. Both joints anteriorly subluxed. Transverse and alar ligaments incompetent.
Type IV: Rare; both joints posteriorly subluxed.
Type V: (Levine and Edwards) frank dislocation; extremely rare.

Fractures of the Odontoid Process (Dens)

Anderson and D'Alonzo Classification (Figure 1.2)
Type I: Oblique avulsion fracture of the apex (5%).
Type II: Fracture at the junction of the body and the neck; high nonunion rate (60%).
Type III: Fracture extends into the body of C2 and may involve the lateral facets (30%).

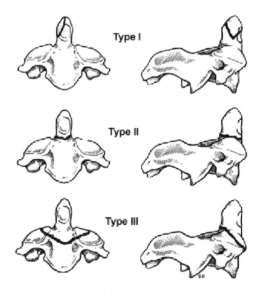

FIGURE 1.2. Anderson and D'Alonzo classification of fractures of the odontoid process (Dens). (Reproduced with permission and copyright © of The Journal of Bone and Joint Surgery, Inc. Anderson LD, d'Alonzo RT. Fractures of the Odontoid process of the axis. *J Bone Joint Surg Am* 1974;56A:1663–1674.)

TRAUMATIC SPONDYLOLISTHESIS OF AXIS (HANGMAN'S FRACTURE)

Levine and Edwards (Figure 1.3)

Type I: Minimally displaced with no angulation; translation <3 mm; stable.

Type II: Significant angulation at C2–C3; translation >3 mm; unstable; C2–C3 disc disrupted. Subclassified into flexion, extension, and listhetic types.

Type IIA: Avulsion of entire C2–C3 intervertebral disc in flexion, leaving the anterior longitudinal ligament intact. Results in severe angulation. No translation; unstable due to flexion-distraction injury.

Type III: Rare; results from initial anterior facet dislocation of C2 on C3 followed by extension injury fracturing the neural arch. Results in severe angulation and translation with unilateral or bilateral facet dislocation of C2–C3; unstable.

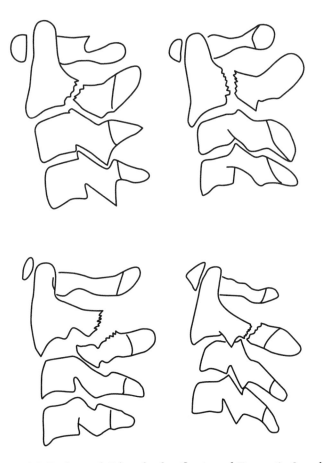

FIGURE 1.3. Levine and Edwards classification of Traumatic Spondylolisthesis of axis: Type I (top left), Type II (top right), Type IIA (bottom left), Type III (bottom right). (Reproduced with permission and copyright © of The Journal of Bone and Joint Surgery, Inc. Levine AM, Edwards CC. The management of traumatic spondylolisthesis of the axis. *J Bone Joint Surg Am* 1985;67A:217–226.)

INJURIES TO C3–C7

Allen Classification
1. Compressive flexion (shear mechanism resulting in "teardrop" fractures)
   Stage I: Blunting of anterior body; posterior element intact.
   Stage II: "Beaking" of the anterior body; loss of anterior vertebral height.

Stage III: Fracture line passing from anterior body through the inferior subchondral plate.

Stage IV: Inferoposterior margin displaced <3 mm into the spinal canal.

Stage V: Teardrop fracture; inferoposterior margin >3 mm into the spinal canal; posterior ligaments and the posterior longitudinal ligament have failed.

2. Vertical compression (burst fractures)

Stage I: Fracture through superior or inferior endplate with no displacement.

Stage II: Fracture through both endplates with minimal displacement.

Stage III: Burst fracture; displacement of fragments peripherally and into the neural canal.

3. Distractive flexion (dislocations)

Stage I: Failure of the posterior ligaments, divergence of spinous processes, and facet subluxation.

Stage II: Unilateral facet dislocation; displacement is always <50%.

Stage III: Bilateral facet dislocation; displacement >50%.

Stage IV: Bilateral facet dislocation with 100% translation.

4. Compressive extension

Stage I: Unilateral vertebral arch fracture.

Stage II: Bilaminar fracture without other tissue failure.

Stage III: Bilateral vertebral arch fracture with fracture of the articular processes, pedicles, and lamina without vertebral body displacement.

Stage IV: Bilateral vertebral arch fracture with full vertebral body displacement anteriorly; ligamentous failure at the posterosuperior and anteroinferior margins.

5. Distractive extension

Stage I: Failure of anterior ligamentous complex or transverse fracture of the body; widening of the disc space and no posterior displacement.

Stage II: Failure of posterior ligament complex with displacement of the vertebral body into the canal.

6. Lateral flexion

Stage I: Asymmetric unilateral compression fracture of the vertebral body plus a vertebral arch fracture on the ipsilateral side without displacement.

Stage II: Displacement of the arch on the anteroposterior view or failure of the ligaments on the contralateral side with articular process separation.

ORTHOPAEDIC TRAUMA ASSOCIATION (OTA) CLASSIFICATION OF CERVICAL SPINE INJURIES

Type A: Compression injuries of the body (compressive forces)

 Type A1: Impaction fractures

 Type A2: Split fractures

 Type A3: Burst fractures

Type B: Distraction injuries of the anterior and posterior elements (tensile forces)

 Type B2: Posterior disruption predominantly osseous (flexion-distraction injury)

 Type B3: Anterior disruption through the disk (hyperextension-shear injury)

Type C: Multidirectional injuries with translation affecting the anterior and posterior elements (axial torque causing rotation injuries)

 Type C1: Rotational wedge, split, and burst fractures

 Type C2: Flexion subluxation with rotation

 Type C3: Rotational shear injuries (Holdsworth slice rotation fracture)

THORACOLUMBAR SPINE FRACTURES

McAfee Classification

Classification is based on the failure mode of the middle osteoligamentous complex (posterior longitudinal ligament, posterior half of the vertebral body, and posterior annulus fibrosus): The six injury patterns are the following:

1. Wedge-compression fracture
2. Stable burst fracture
3. Unstable burst fracture
4. Chance fracture
5. Flexion-distraction injury
6. Translational injuries

Denis Classification

The three-column model according to Denis (Figure 1.4):

Anterior Column:
 Anterior longitudinal ligament
 Anterior half of vertebral body
 Anterior portion of annulus fibrosis

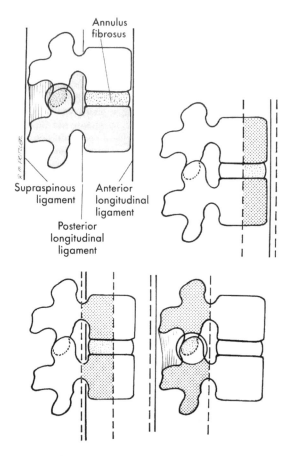

FIGURE 1.4. Denis' concept of three-column model.

Middle column:
  Posterior longitudinal ligament
  Posterior half of vertebral body
  Posterior aspect of annulus fibrosis
Posterior column:
  Neural arch
  Ligamentum flavum
  Facet capsule
  Interspinous ligament

TABLE 1.1. Pattern of failure.

	Column		
Type	Anterior	Middle	Posterior
1. Compression	Compression	none	none/distraction
2. Burst	Compression	Compression	None/Splaying of pedicles
3. Flexion-Distraction	None/Distraction	Distraction	distraction
4. Flexion-Dislocation	Compression/ Rotation/shear	Compression/ Rotation/shear	Compression Rotation/shear

Based on the three-column model, fractures are classified according to the mechanism of injury and the resulting fracture pattern into one of the following categories (see Table 1.1):

1. Compression
2. Burst
3. Flexion-Distraction
4. Fracture-Dislocation

1. Compression Fractures
Four subtypes described on the basis of endplate involvement are as follows:
Type A: Fracture of both endplates
Type B: Fractures of the superior endplate
Type C: Fractures of the inferior endplate
Type D: Both endplates intact

2. Burst Fractures (Figure 1.5)
Type A: Fractures of both endplates
Type B: Fracture of the superior endplate
Type C: Fracture of the inferior endplate
Type D: Burst rotation
Type E: Burst lateral flexion

3. Flexion-Distraction Injuries (Chance Fractures, Seat Belt-Type Injuries)
Type A: One-level bony injury
Type B: One-level ligamentous
Type C: Two-level injury through bony middle column
Type D: Two-level injury through ligamentous middle column

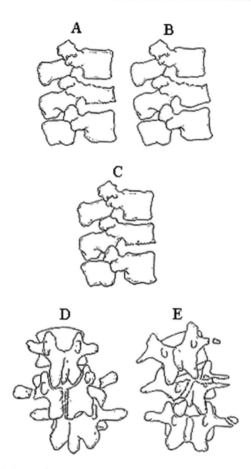

FIGURE 1.5. Burst thoracolumbar spine fractures.

4. Fracture Dislocations

Type A: Flexion-rotation. Posterior and middle column fail in tension and rotation; anterior column fails in compression and rotation; 75% have neurological deficits, 52% of these are complete lesions.

Type B: Shear. Shear failure of all three columns, most commonly in the postero-anterior direction; all cases with complete neurological deficits.

Type C: Flexion-distraction. Tension failure of posterior and middle columns, with anterior tear of annulus fibrosus and stripping of the anterior longitudinal ligament; 75% with neurological deficits (all incomplete).

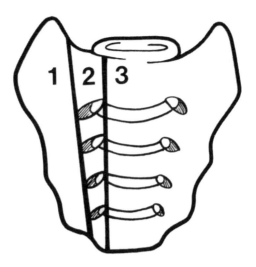

FIGURE 1.6. Denis classification of sacral fractures.

SACRAL FRACTURES (Figure 1.6)

Denis Classification

Zone 1: the region of the ala
Zone 2: the region of the sacral foramina
Zone 3: the region of central sacral canal

Chapter 2
Shoulder and Upper Limb

CLAVICLE

Craig Classification

Group I: Fracture of the middle third

Group II: Fracture of the distal third. Subclassified according to the location of coracoclavicular ligaments relative to the fracture as follows:

 Type I: Minimal displacement: interligamentous fracture between conoid and trapezoid or between the coracoclavicular and acromiocavicular ligaments

 Type II: Displaced secondary to a fracture medial to the coracoclavicular ligaments – higher incidence of non-union

 IIA: Conoid and trapezoid attached to the distal segment (see Figure 2.1)

 IIB: Conoid torn, trapezoid attached to the distal segment (see Figure 2.2)

 Type III: Fracture of the articular surface of the acromioclavicular joint with no ligamentous injury – may be confused with first-degree acromioclavicular joint separation

Group III: Fracture of the proximal third:

 Type I: Minimal displacement

 Type II: Significant displaced (ligamentous rupture)

 Type III: Intraarticular

 Type IV: Epiphyseal separation

 Type V: Comminuted

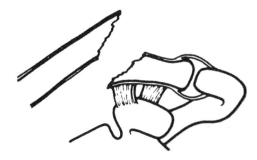

FIGURE 2.1. Type IIA clavicular fracture according to Craig classification. (Reprinted from Craig EV. Fractures of the clavicle in Rockwood CA, Matsen FA (eds): *The shoulder*. Philadelphia, Saunders © 1990, with permission from Elsevier.)

Acromioclavicular Joint

Rockwood Classification (Figure 2.3)

Type I
- Sprain of the acromioclavicular (AC) ligament.
- AC joint tenderness, minimal pain with arm motion, no pain in coracoclavicular interspaces.
- No abnormality on radiographs.

Type II
- AC ligament tear with joint disruption and sprained coracoclavicular ligaments. Distal clavicle is slightly superior to acromion and mobile to palpation; tenderness is found in the coracoclavicular space.

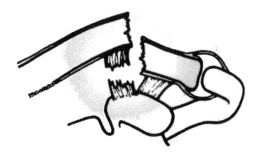

FIGURE 2.2. Type IIB clavicular fracture according to Craig classification. (Reprinted from Craig EV. Fractures of the clavicle in Rockwood CA, Matsen FA (eds): *The shoulder*. Philadelphia, Saunders © 1990, with permission from Elsevier.)

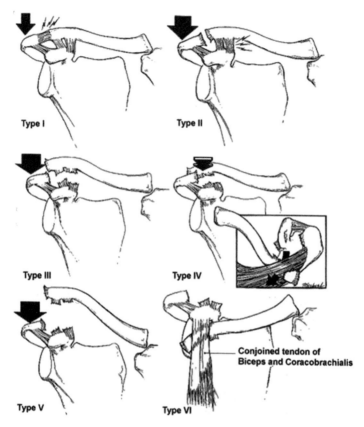

FIGURE 2.3. Types I–VI of the Rockwood classification for acromioclavicular joints. (Reproduced from Heckman JD, Bucholz RW (Eds). Rockwood, Green and Wilkins' Fractures in Adults, Philadelphia: 2001.)

■ Radiographs demonstrate slight elevation of the distal end of the clavicle and AC joint widening. Stress films show the coracoclavicular ligaments are sprained but integrity is maintained.

Type III

■ AC and coracoclavicular ligaments torn with AC joint dislocation; deltoid and trapezius muscles usually detached from the distal clavicle.

■ The upper extremity and distal fragment are depressed, and the distal end of the proximal fragment may tent the skin. The AC joint is tender, coracoclavicular widening is evident.

■ Radiographs demonstrate the distal clavicle superior to the medial border of the acromion; stress views reveal a widened coracoclavicular interspace 25% to 100% greater than the normal side.

Type IV

■ Type III with the distal clavicle displaced posteriorly into or through the trapezius.

■ Clinically, more pain exists than in type III; the distal clavicle is displaced posteriorly away from the clavicle.

■ Axillary radiograph or computed tomography demonstrates posterior displacement of the distal clavicle.

Type V

■ Type III with the distal clavicle grossly and severely displaced superiorly.

■ This type is typically associated with tenting of the skin.

■ Radiographs demonstrate the coracoclavicular interspace to be 100% to 300% greater than the normal side.

Type VI

■ AC dislocated, with the clavicle displaced inferior to the acromion or the coracoid; the coracoclavicular interspace is decreased compared with normal.

■ The deltoid and trapezius muscles are detached from the distal clavicle.

■ The mechanism of injury is usually a severe direct force onto the superior surface of the distal clavicle, with abduction of the arm and scapula retraction.

■ Clinically, the shoulder has a flat appearance with a prominent acromion; associated clavicle and upper rib fractures and brachial plexus injuries are due to high energy trauma.

■ Radiographs demonstrate one of two types of inferior dislocation: subacromial or subcoracoid.

Sternoclavicular Joint

Anatomic Classification

Anterior dislocation – more common
Posterior dislocation

Etiologic Classification

Sprain or subluxation
 Mild: joint stable, ligamentous integrity maintained.
 Moderate: subluxation, with partial ligamentous disruption.
 Severe: unstable joint, with complete ligamentous compromise.

SCAPULA

Zdravkovic and Damholt Classification
Type I: Scapula body
Type II: Apophyseal fractures, including the acromion and coracoid
Type III: Fractures of the superolateral angle, including the scapular neck and glenoid

Coracoid Fractures

Eyres and Brooks Classification (Figure 2.4)
Type I: Coracoid tip or epiphyseal fracture
Type II: Mid process

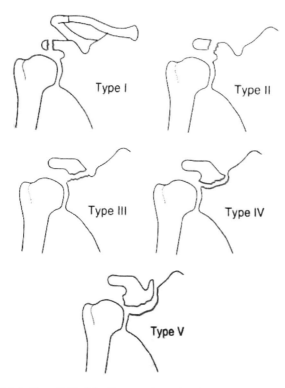

FIGURE 2.4. Types I–V of the Eyres and Brooks classification for coracoid fractures. (Reproduced with permission and copyright © of the British Editorial Society of Bone and Joint Surgery. Eyre KS, Brook A, Stanley D. Fractures of coracoid process. *J Bone Joint Surg* 1995;77B:425–428.)

Type III: Basal fracture
Type IV: Involvement of superior body of scapula
Type V: Extension into the glenoid fossa

The suffix of A or B can be used to record the presence of absence of damage to the clavicle or its ligamentous connection to the scapula.

Intraarticular Glenoid Fractures

Ideberg Classification (Figure 2.5)
Type I: Avulsion fracture of the anterior margin.
Type II

> Type IIA: Transverse fracture through the glenoid fossa exiting inferiorly.
>
> Type IIB: Oblique fracture through the glenoid fossa exiting inferiorly.

Type III: Oblique fracture through the glenoid exiting superiorly; often associated with an acromioclavicular joint injury.
Type IV: Transverse fracture exiting through the medial border of the scapula.
Type V: Combination of a Type II and Type IV pattern.
Type VI: Severe continuation of glenoid surface (GOSS).

Anterior Glenohumeral Dislocations

Classification
Degree of instability:
Dislocation/subluxation
Chronology/Type
  Congenital
  Acute versus chronic
  Locked (fixed)
  Recurrent
Force
  Atraumatic
  Traumatic
Patient contribution: voluntary /involuntary
Direction
  Subcoracoid
  Subglenoid
  Intrathoracic

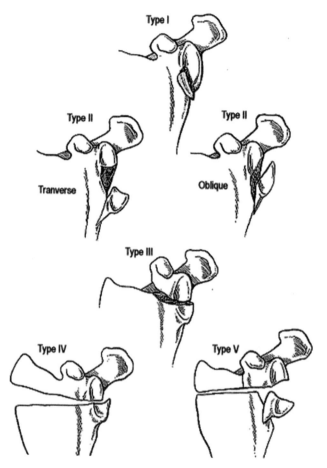

FIGURE 2.5. Ideberg classification of intraarticular glenoid fractures. Ideberg R. Fractures of the scapula involving the glenoid fossa. (From Batemans JE, Welsh RP (eds): In *The surgery of the shoulder*. Philadelphia, Decker 1984:63–66.)

Posterior Glenohumeral Dislocation

Anatomic Classification

Subacromial (98%): Articular surface directed posteriorly; the lesser tuberosity typically occupies the glenoid fossa; often associated with an impaction fracture on the anterior humeral head.

Subglenoid (very rare): Humeral head posterior and inferior to the glenoid.

Subspinous (very rare): Humeral head medial to the acromion and inferior to the spine of the scapula.

Inferior Glenohumeral Dislocation (Luxatio Erecta)

Superiod Glenohumeral Dislocation

Proximal Humerus

Neer Classification (Figure 2.6)

■ The four parts are the greater and lesser tuberosities, the shaft, and the humeral head.

■ A part is displaced if >1 cm of displacement or >45 degree of angulation is seen.

At least two views of the proximal humerus (anteroposterior and scapular Y views) must be obtained; additionally, the axillary view is very helpful for ruling out dislocation.

Humeral Shaft

Descriptive Classification

Open/closed

Location: proximal third, middle third, distal third

Degree: incomplete, complete

Direction and character: transverse, oblique, spiral, segmental, comminuted

Intrinsic condition of the bone

Articular extension

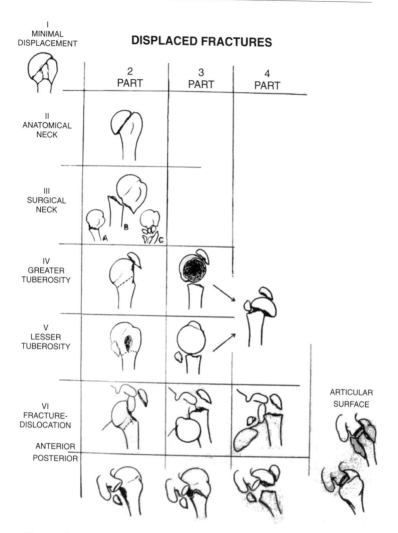

FIGURE 2.6. Neer classification of fractures to the proximal humerus. (Reproduced with permission and copyright © of The Journal of Bone and Joint Surgery, Inc. Neer, CS. Displaced Proximal Humeral Fractures: I. Classification and Evaluation. *J Bone Joint Surg* 1970;52A:1077–1089.)

AO Classification of Humeral Diaphyseal Fractures (Figure 2.7)

Type A: Simple fracture
          A1: Spiral
          A2: Oblique (>30°)
          A3: Transverse (<30°)
Type B: Wedge fracture
          B1: Spiral wedge
          B2: Bending wedge
          B3: Fragmented wedge
Type C: Complex fracture
          C1: Spiral
          C2: Segmented
          C3: Irregular (significant comminution)

Distal Humerus

Descriptive

Supracondylar fractures: Extension type or flexion type
Transcondylar fractures: The fracture passes through both condyles and is within the joint capsule

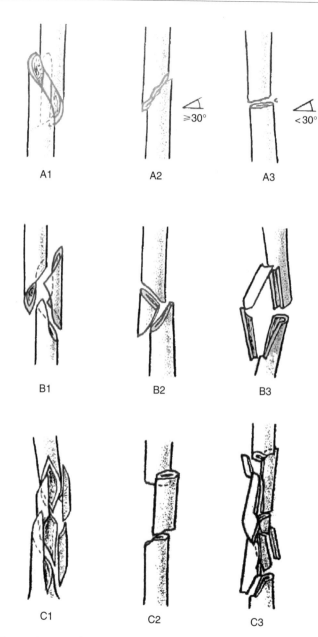

FIGURE 2.7. AO classification of humeral diaphyseal fractures.

Intercondylar Fractures

Riseborough and Radin Classification (Figure 2.8)

Type I: Nondisplaced

Type II: Slight displacement with no rotation between the condylar fragments in the frontal plane

Type III: Displacement with rotation

Type IV: Severe comminution of the articular surface

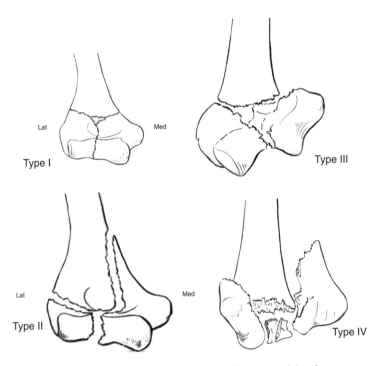

FIGURE 2.8. Type I, Type II, Type III, Type IV intercondylar fractures. (Reproduced with permission and copyright © from The Journal of Bone and Joint Surgery, Inc. Riseborough EJ, Radin EL, Intercondylar T fractures of the humerus in the adult. A comparison of operative and non-operative treatment in twenty-nine cases. *J Bone Joint Surg* 1969;51A:130–141.)

Condylar Fractures

Milch Classification (Figure 2.9)

Two types for medial and lateral; the key is the lateral trochlear ridge.

Type I: Lateral trochlear ridge is left intact.
Type II: Lateral trochlear ridge is part of the condylar fragment (medial or lateral).
          Medial
          Lateral

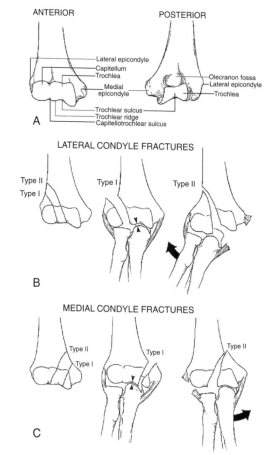

FIGURE 2.9. Milch classification of condylar fractures. (Milch H. Fractures and fracture-dislocations of the humeral condyles. *J Trauma* 1964;4:592–607.)

CAPITELLUM FRACTURES

Classification (Figure 2.10)

Type I: Hahn-Steinthal fragment. Large osseous component of capitellum, sometimes with trochlear involvement

Type II: Kocher-Lorenz fragment. Articular cartilage with minimal subchondral bone attached: "uncapping of the condyle"

Type III: Markedly comminuted

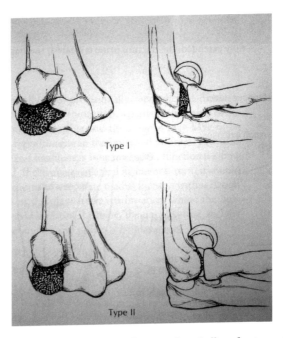

FIGURE 2.10. Types I and II classification of capitellum fractures. (From Hahn NF. Fall von Cine Besonderes Varietat der Frakturen des Ellenbogens. Z *Wundarzte Geburtshilfe* 1853;6:185–189. Steinthal D. Die isolierte Fraktur der Eminentia capitata in Ellenbogengelenk. *Zentralbl Chir* 1898;15:17–20. Kocher T. Beitrage zur Kenntniss Einiger Tisch Wichtiger Frakturformen. Basel, Sallman, 1896:585–591. Lorenz H. Zur Kenntniss der Fractura humeri (eminentiae capitatae). *Dtsch Z Chir* 1905;78:531–545. Reproduced from Heckman JD, Bucholz RW (Eds), Rockwood, Green, and Wilkins' Fractures in Adults. Philadelphia: 2001.)

CORONOID PROCESS FRACTURE

Regan and Morrey classification (Figure 2.11)

Type I: Fracture avulsion just the tip of the coronoid

Type II: Those that involve less than 50% of coronoid either as single fracture or multiple fragments

Type III: Those involve >50% of coronoid

Subdivided into those without (A) and with elbow dislocation (B)

OLECRANON

Morrey Classification

Type I: Undisplaced, stable fractures

Type II: Displaced, stable

Type III: Displaced, unstable fractures

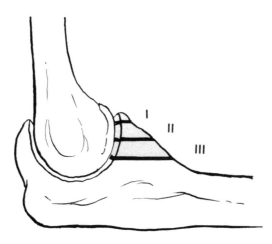

FIGURE 2.11. Regan and Morrey classification of coronoid process fractures. (Reproduced with permission and copyright © of The Journal of Bone and Joint Surgery, Inc. Regan W, Morrey B. Fracture of coronoid process of the ulna. *J Bone Joint Surg* 1989;71-A:1348–1354.)

RADIAL HEAD

Mason Classification (Figure 2.12)

Type I: Nondisplaced marginal fractures

Type II: Marginal fractures with displacement (impaction, depression, angulation)

Type III: Comminuted fractures involving the entire head

Type IV: Associated with dislocation of the elbow (Johnston)

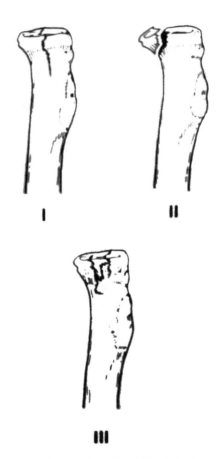

FIGURE 2.12. Mason classification of radial head fractures. (From Mason ML. Some observations on fractures of the head of the radius with a review of one hundred cases. *Br J Surg* 1954;42:123–132.)

ELBOW DISLOCATION

Classification (Figure 2.13)

Chronology: acute, chronic (unreduced), recurrent

Descriptive: based on relationship of radius/ulna to the distal humerus, as follows:

- Posterior
  Posterolateral: >90% dislocations
  Posteromedial
- Anterior
- Lateral
- Medial
- Divergent (rare)
  *Anterior-posterior type (ulna posterior, radial head anterior).
  *Mediolateral (transverse) type (distal humerus wedged between radius lateral and ulna medial).

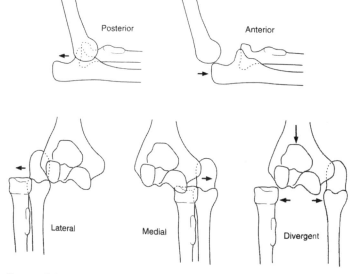

FIGURE 2.13. Classification of elbow dislocation.

FOREARM

Descriptive Classification
- Closed versus open
- Location
- Comminuted, segmental, or multifragmented
- Displacement
- Angulation
- Rotational alignment

Monteggia Fractures (Figure 2.14)
Fracture of the shaft of the ulna with associated dislocation of the radial head.

Bado Classification
Type I: Anterior dislocation of the radial head with fracture of the ulnar diaphysis at any level with anterior angulation.

Type II: Posterior/posterolateral dislocation of the radial head with fracture of the ulnar diaphysis with posterior angulation.

Type III: Pateral/anterolateral dislocation of the radial head with fracture of the ulnar metaphysic.

Type IV: Anterior dislocation of the radial head with fractures of both the radius and ulna within proximal third at the same level.

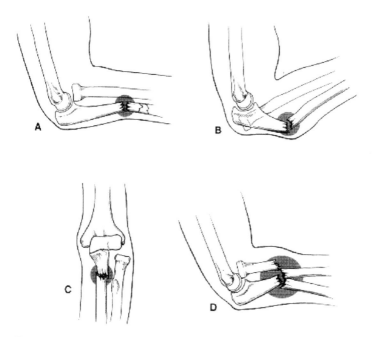

FIGURE 2.14. Monteggia fractures. (Reproduced with permission from Lippincott Williams & Wilkins. Bado JL. The Monteggia lesion. *Clin Orthop* 1967;50:70–86.)

TABLE 2.1. Frykman classification of distal radius.

	Distal ulnar fracture	
Fracture	Absent	Present
Extraarticular	I	II
Intraarticular involving radiocarpal joint	III	IV
Intraarticular involving distal radioulnar joint	V	VI
Intraarticular involving radiocarpal and distal radioulnar joint	VII	VIII

DISTAL RADIUS

Descriptive Classification (Table 2.1 and Figure 2.15)
- Open/closed
- Displacement
- Angulation

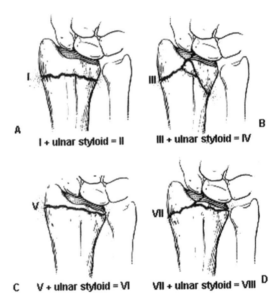

FIGURE 2.15. Fractures of the distal radius. (From Frykman G. Fracture of the distal radius including sequelae – shoulder-hand-finger ayndrome, disturbance in the distal radio-ulnar joint, and impairment of nerve function: a clinical and experimental study. *Acta Orthop Scand* 1967; 108(Suppl.):1–153. Reproduced with permission from Taylor and Francis Ltd.)

- Comminution
- Loss of radial length
- Intraarticular involvement

SMITH FRACTURE

Modified Thomas' Classification (Figure 2.16)
Type I: Extra articular
Type II: Fracture line crosses into the dorsal articular surface
Type III: Fracture line enters the carpal joint (Volar Barton)

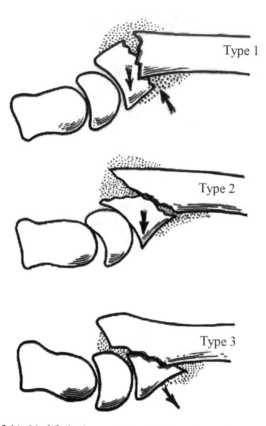

FIGURE 2.16. Modified Thomas' classification. (Reproduced with permission and copyright © of the British Editorial Society of Bone and Joint Surgery. Thomas FB. Reduction of Smith's fracture. *J Bone Joint Surg* 1957;39B:463–470.)

SCAPHOID FRACTURES

Russe classification
1. Horizontal oblique
   Distal third
   Middle third (waist)
   Proximal third
2. Transverse fracture line
3. Vertical oblique fracture line

Herbert and Fisher Classification (Figure 2.17)
Type A: Acute Stable fractures
       Type A1: Fracture of tubercle
       Type A2: Undisplaced "crack" fracture of the waist
Type B: Acute Unstable fractures
       Type B1: Oblique fractures of distal third
       Type B2: Displaced or mobile fracture of the waist
       Type B3: Proximal pole fractures
       Type B4: Fracture dislocation of carpus
       Type B5: Comminuted fractures
Type C: Delayed union
Type D: Established nonunion
       Type D1: Fibrous non-union
       Type D2: Sclerotic nonunion (Pseudoarthrosis)

Note that stable indicates nondisplaced fractures with no step-off in any plane; unstable indicates displacement with 1 mm or more step-off with scapholunate angulation >60 degrees or lunatocapitate angulation >15 degrees.

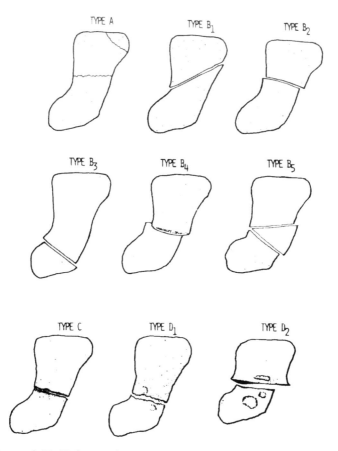

FIGURE 2.17. Herbert and Fisher classification. (Reproduced with permission and copyright © of the British Editorial Society of Bone and Joint Surgery. Herbert T, Fisher W. Management of the fractured scaphoid using a new bone screw. *J Bone Joint Surg* 1984;66B,114–123.)

LUNATE FRACTURES

Teisen and Hjarkbaek Classification (Figure 2.18)

Group I: Fracture volar pole, possibly affecting the volar nutrient artery

Group II: Chip fracture which does not affect the main blood supply

Group III: Fracture of dorsal pole of the Lunate possibly affecting the blood supply

Group IV: Sagittal fracture through the body of Lunate

Group V: Transverse fractures through the body of the Lunate

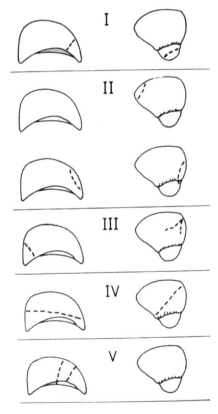

FIGURE 2.18. Teisen and Hjarbaek classification. Left: lateral view; right: AP view. (Teisen and Hjarbaek, Classification of fresh fractures. *J Hand Surg* 13(B):458–462. Copyright 1988 The British Society for Surgery of the hand. With permission from Elsevier.)

THUMB

Intraarticular Fractures (Figure 2.19)

Type I: Bennett fracture – fracture line separates major part of metacarpal from volar lip fragment, producing a disruption of the first carpometacarpal joint; first metacarpal is pulled proximally by the abductor pollicis longus.

Type II: Rolando fracture – requires greater force than a Bennett fracture; presently used to describe a comminuted Bennett fracture, a "Y" or "T" fracture, or a fracture with dorsal and palmar fragments.

Extraarticular fractures

Type IIIA: Transverse fracture
Type IIIB: Oblique fracture
Type IV: Epiphyseal injuries seen in children.

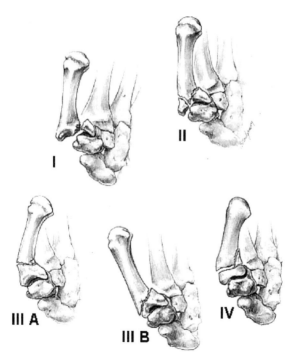

FIGURE 2.19. Intraarticular fractures of the thumb. (From Green DP, O'Brien ET. Fractures of the thumb metacarpal. *South Med J* 1972;65:807. Permission requested from Lippincott Williams & Wilkins.)

Type I

Type II

Type III

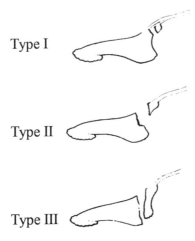

FIGURE 2.20. Wehbe and Schneider classification. (Reproduced with permission and copyright © from The Journal of Bone and Joint Surgery, Inc. Wehbe MA, Schneider LH. Mallet fractures. *J Bone Joint Surg* 1984;66-A:658–669.)

DISTAL PHALANX FRACTURES

Kaplan Classification
Type I: Longitudinal split
Type II: Comminuted tuft
Type III: Transverse fracture

MALLET FRACTURE

Wehbe and Schneider classification (Figure 2.20)
Type I: Mallet fractures including bone injuries of varying extend without subluxation of distal interphalangyal joint
Type II: Fractures are associated with subluxation distal interphalangyal joint
Type III: Epiphyseal and physeal injuries. Each type then divided into three subtypes:
   Type IIIA: Fracture fragment involving less than one-third of articular surface of distal phalanx
   Type IIIB: A fracture fragment involving one-third to two-thirds of articular surface
   Type IIIC: A fragment that involves more than two-thirds of articular surface

Chapter 3
Pelvis and Lower Limb

PELVIS

Young and Burgess Classification (Figure 3.1)
1. Lateral compression
2. Anteroposterior compression
3. Vertical shear
4. Combined mechanical

Description:
1. Lateral compression (LC): Transverse fractures of the pubic rami, ipsilateral, or contralateral to posterior injury
   Type I: Sacral compression on the side of impact
   Type II: Posterior iliac wing fracture (crescent) on the side of impact
   Type III: LCI or LCII injury on the side of impact; contralateral open book injury
2. Anteroposterior compression: Symphyseal diastasis or longitudinal rami fractures
   Type I: <2.5 cm of symphyseal diastasis; vertical fractures of one or both pubic rami intact posterior ligaments
   Type II: <2.5 cm of symphyseal diastasis; widening of sacroiliac joint due to anterior sacroiliac ligament disruption; disruption of the sacrotuberous, sacrospinous, and symphyseal ligaments with intact posterior sacroiliac ligaments result in "open book" injury with internal and external rotational instability; vertical stability is maintained
   Type III: Complete disruption of the symphysis, sacrotuberous, sacrospinous, and sacroiliac ligaments resulting in extreme rotational instability and lateral displacement; no cephaloposterior displacement; completely unstable with the highest rate of associated neurovascular injuries and blood loss

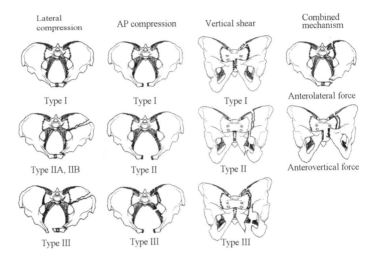

Lateral compression — AP compression — Vertical shear — Combined mechanism

Type I — Type I — Type I — Anterolateral force

Type IIA, IIB — Type II — Type II — Anterovertical force

Type III — Type III — Type III

FIGURE 3.1. Young and Burgess classification of pelvic ring fractures. (From Young JWR, Burgess AR. *Radiologic management of pelvic ring fractures*. Baltimore, Urban & Schwarzenberg, 1987.)

3. Vertical shear: symphyseal diastasis or vertical displaced anterior and posterior usually through the SI joint, occasionally through the iliac wing or sacrum.
4. Combined mechanical: combination of injuries often due to crush mechanisms; most common is vertical shear and lateral compression.

Tile Classification
Type A: Stable
 Type A1: Fractures of the pelvis not involving the ring; avulsion injuries
 Type A2: Stable, minimally displaced fractures of the ring
Type B: Rotationally unstable, vertically stable.
 Type B1: Open-book
 Type B2: Lateral compression; ipsilateral
 Type B3: Lateral compression; contralateral (bucket handle)
Type C: Rotationally and vertically unstable.
 Type C1: Unilateral.

Type C2: Bilateral; one side rotationally unstable, with
contralateral side vertically Unstable.
Type C3: Associated acetabular fracture.

Acetabulum

Judet-Letournel Classification (Figure 3.2)

Elementary patterns   Associated patterns
1. Posterior wall   1. T-shaped
2. Posterior column   2. Posterior column and posterior wall
3. Anterior wall   3. Transverse and posterior wall
4. Anterior column   4. Anterior column:
5. Transverse   Posterior
                              Hemitransverse
                           5. Both columns

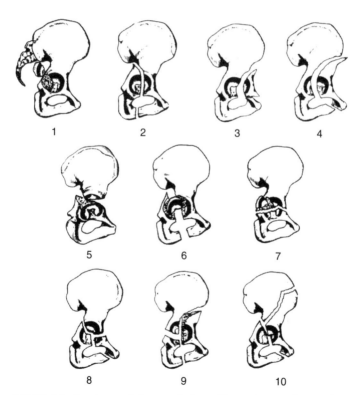

FIGURE 3.2. Fractures of the acetabulum. (From Letournel E, Judet R.
Fractures of the acetabulum. New York, Springer-Verlag, 1981. With kind
permission of Springer Science, Business & Media.)

HIP DISLOCATIONS: ANTERIOR DISLOCATIONS
Inferior (obturator) dislocation
Superior (iliac or pubic) dislocation

Epstein Classification of Anterior Dislocations of the Hip
(Figure 3.3)

Type I: Superior dislocations, including pubic and subspinous

    Type IA: No associated fractures

    Type IB: Associated fracture or impaction of the femoral head

    Type IC: Associated fracture of the acetabulum

Type II: Inferior dislocations, including obturator and perineal

    Type IIA: No associated fractures

    Type IIB: Associated fractures or impaction of the femoral head/neck

    Type IIC: Associated fracture of the acetabulum

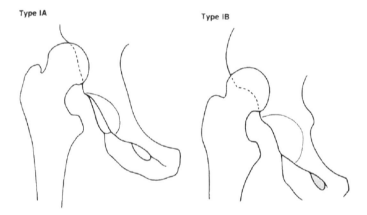

FIGURE 3.3. Epstein classification of anterior dislocations of the hip.

Type IC

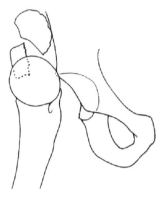

Type IIA

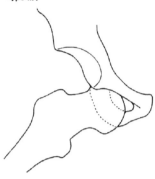

Type IIB

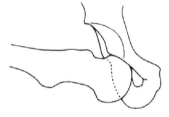

Type IIC

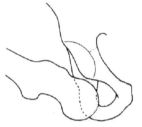

FIGURE 3.3. *Continued*

HIP DISLOCATIONS: POSTERIOR DISLOCATION

Thompson and Epstein Classification of Posterior Dislocations of the Hip (Figure 3.4)

Type I: Dislocation with or without an insignificant posterior wall fragment

Type II: Dislocation associated with a single large posterior wall fragment

Type III: Dislocation with a comminuted posterior wall fragment

Type IV: Dislocation with fracture of the acetabular floor

Type V: Dislocation with fracture of the femoral head

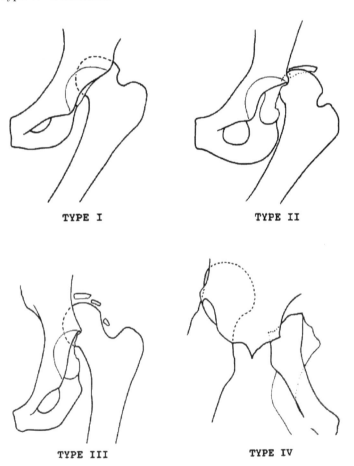

TYPE I   TYPE II

TYPE III   TYPE IV

FIGURE 3.4. Thompson and Epstein classification of posterior dislocations of the hip.

Femoral Head

The Thompson & Epstein type V fracture dislocation has been subclassified into four types:

Pipkin Subclassification (Figure 3.5)

Type I: Posterior hip dislocation with fracture of the femoral head inferior to the fovea centralis.

Type II: Posterior hip dislocation with fracture of the femoral head superior to the fovea centralis.

Type III: Type II injury or I associated with fracture of the femoral neck.

Type IV: Type I, II, or III associated with fracture of the acetabular rim.

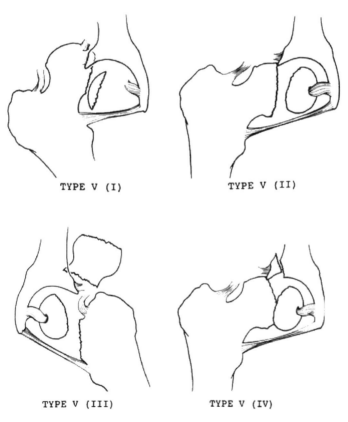

FIGURE 3.5. Pipkin classification of femoral head fractures. (From Hansen S, Swiontkowski M. *Orthopedic trauma protocols*. New York, Raven Press, 1993:238.)

Femoral Neck Fractures

Classification by Anatomic Location
■ Subcapital
■ Transcervical
■ Basocervical

Pauwels Classification (Figure 3.6)
Based on angle of fracture from horizontal plane:

Type I: 30°
Type II: 50°
Type III: 70°

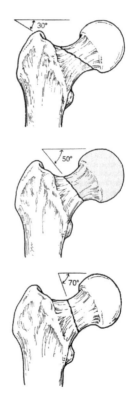

FIGURE 3.6. Pauwels classification of femoral neck fractures.

Garden Classification (Figure 3.7)

Based on degree of valgus displacement.

Stage I: Incomplete/impacted.

Stage II: Complete nondisplaced on anteroposterior and lateral views.

Stage III: Complete with partial displacement; trabecular pattern of the femoral head does not line up with that of the acetabulum.

Stage IV: Completely displaced; trabecular pattern of the head assumes a parallel orientation with that of the acetabulum.

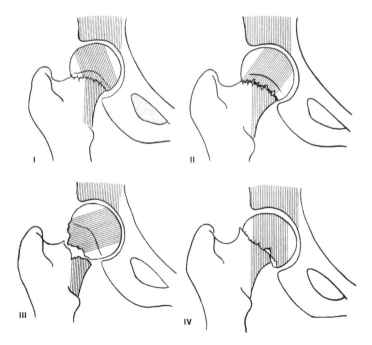

FIGURE 3.7. Garden classification of femoral neck fractures. (From Garden RS. Low angle fracture of the femoral neck. *J Bone Joint Surg* 1961;3-B;674–663.)

Intertrochanteric Fractures

Boyd and Griffin Classification (Figure 3.8)

Type I: A single fracture along the intertrochanteric line, stable and easily reducible.

Type II: Major fracture line along the intertrochanteric line with comminution in the coronal plane.

Type III: Fracture at the level of the lesser trochanter with variable comminution and extension into the subtrochanteric region (reverse obliquity).

Type IV: Fracture extending into the proximal femoral shaft in at least two planes.

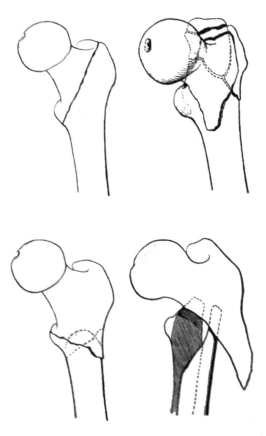

FIGURE 3.8. The Boyd and Griffin classification of trochanteric fractures: Type I (top left), Type II (top right), Type III (bottom left), Type IV (bottom right). (From Boyd HB, Griffin LL. Classification and treatment of trochanteric fractures. *Arch Surg* 1949;58:853–866.)

Evans Classification (Figure 3.9)

Type I:

> Stable:
> - Undisplaced fractures.
> - Displaced but after reduction overlap of the medial cortical buttress make the fracture stable.
>
> Unstable:
> - Displaced and the medial cortical buttress is not restored by reduction of fracture.
> - Displaced and comminuted fractures in which the medial cortical buttress is not restored by reduction of the fracture.

Type II: Reverse obliquity fractures.

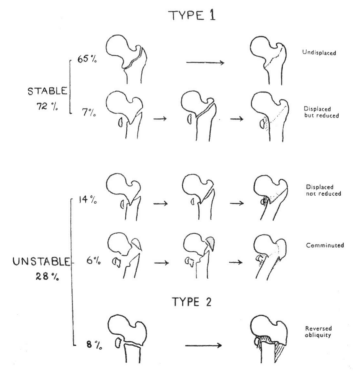

FIGURE 3.9. Trochanteric fractures. (Reproduced with permission and copyright © of the British Editorial Society of Bone and Joint Surgery. Ewans EM. The treatment of trochanteric fractures of the femur. *J Bone Joint Surg* 1949;31-B:190–203.)

Subtrochanteric Fractures

Fielding Classification (Figure 3.10)

Based on the location of the primary fracture line in relation to the lesser trochanter.

Type I: At level of the lesser trochanter
Type II: <2.5 cm below the lesser trochanter
Type III: 2.5 cm to 5 cm below the lesser trochanter

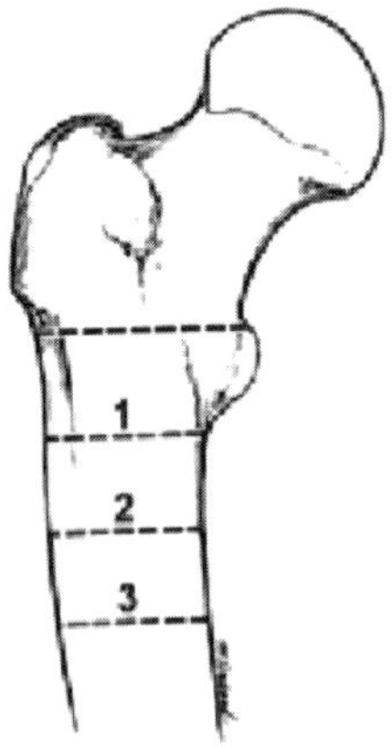

FIGURE 3.10. Fielding classification of subtrochanteric fractures. (From Fielding JW, Magliato HJ. Subtrochanteric fractures. *Surg Gynecol Obstet* 1966;122:555–560, now *J Am Coll Surg*. With Permission from the Journals of American College of Surgeons.)

Seinsheimer Classification (Figure 3.11)

The Seinsheimer classification is based on the number of major bone fragments and the location and shape of the fracture lines.

Type I: Nondisplaced fracture or any fracture with <2 mm of displacement of the fracture fragments.

Type II: Two-part fractures.
           Type IIA: Two-part transverse femoral fracture.
           Type IIB: Two-part spiral fracture with the lesser trochanter attached to the proximal fragment.
           Type IIC: Two-part spiral fracture with the lesser trochanter attached to the distal fragment.

Type III: Three-part fractures.
           Type IIIA: Three-part spiral fracture in which the lesser trochanter is part of the third fragment, which has an inferior spike of cortex of varying length.
           Type IIIB: Three-part spiral fracture of the proximal third of the femur, where the third part is a butterfly fragment.

Type IV: Comminuted fracture with four or more fragments.

Type V: Subtrochanteric-intertrochanteric fracture, including any subtrochanteric fracture with extension through the greater trochanter.

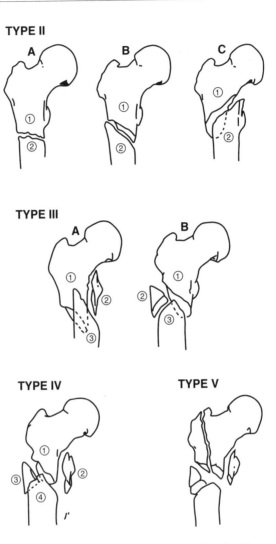

FIGURE 3.11. Seinsheimer classification. (Reproduced with permission and copyright © of The Journal of Bone and Joint Surgery, Inc. Seinsheimer F. Subtrochanteric fractures of the femur. *J Bone Joint Surg* 1977;60-A;300–306.)

Russel-Taylor Classification (Figure 3.12)

Type I: Fractures do not extend into piriformis fossa:

> Type IA: Lesser trochanter is attached to the proximal fragment
>
> Type IB: Lesser trochanter is detached from the proximal fragment

Type II: Fractures that extend into the piriformis fossa:

> Type IIA: No significant comminution or fracture of lesser trochanter
>
> Type IIB: Significant comminution of the medial femoral cortex and loss of continuity of lesser trochanter

Femoral Shaft

Descriptive Classification

- Open versus closed
- Location: proximal, middle, or distal one-third; supraisthmal or infraisthmal
- Pattern: spiral, oblique, or transverse
- Angulation: varus, valgus, or rotational deformity
- Displacement: shortening or translation
- Comminuted, segmental, or butterfly fragment

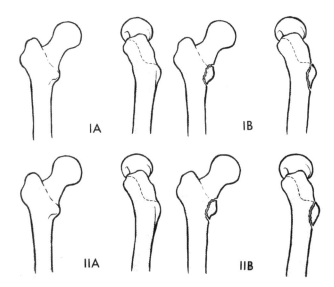

FIGURE 3.12. Russel-Taylor classification.

Winquist and Hansen Classification (Figure 3.13)

The Winquist and Hansen classification is based on comminution; most useful for determining the need for interlocking nails.

Type I: Minimal or no comminution

Type II: Cortices of both fragments at least 50% intact

Type III: 50% to 100% cortical comminution

Type IV: Circumferential comminution with no cortical contact at the fracture site

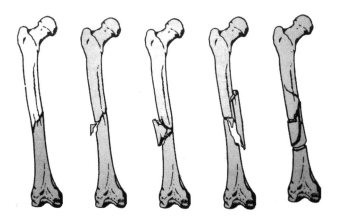

FIGURE 3.13. Winquist and Hansen classification of femoral shaft fractures: from left to right (Type 0, Type I, Type II, Type III, Type IV). (Reproduced with permission from Lippincott Williams & Wilkins. Winquist RA, Hansen ST. Comminuted fractures of the femoral shaft treated by interamedullary nailing. *Orthop Clin* 1980;11;663–648.)

Distal Femur

Descriptive Classification
- Open versus closed
- Location: supracondylar, intercondylar, condylar involvement
- Pattern: spiral, oblique, or transverse
- Articular involvement
- Angulation: varus, valgus, or rotational deformity
- Displacement: shortening or translation
- Comminuted, segmental, or butterfly fragment

AO Classification (Figure 3.14)
Type A: Extra articular
  Type A1: Simple, two-part supracondylar fracture
  Type A2: Metaphyseal wedge
  Type A3: Comminuted supracondylar fracture
Type B: Unicondylar
  Type B1: Lateral condyle, sagittal
  Type B2: Medial condyle, sagittal
  Type B3: Coronal
Type C: Bicondylar
  Type C1: Noncomminuted supracondylar "T" or "Y" fracture
  Type C2: Comminuted supracondylar fracture
  Type C3: Comminuted supracondylar and intercondylar fracture

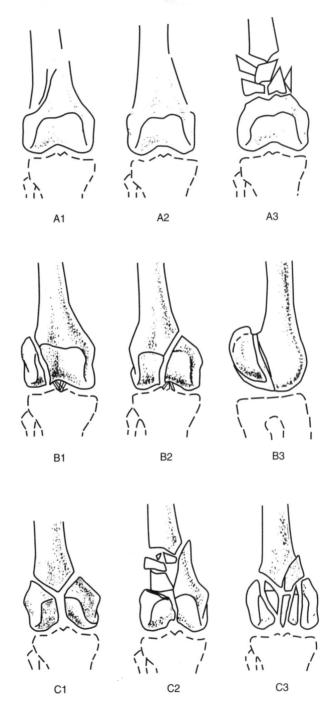

FIGURE 3.14. Classification of the distal femur.

PATELLAR FRACTURES

Descriptive Classification
■ Open versus closed
■ Displacement
■ Pattern: Stellate, comminuted, transverse, vertical (marginal), polar
■ Osteochondral

Saunders Classification (Figure 3.15)
Undisplaced
■ Stellate
■ Transverse
■ Vertical

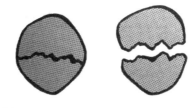

Undisplaced Transverse

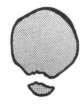

**Lower or
Upper Pole**

Comminuted   Vertical

FIGURE 3.15. Saunders classification.

Displaced
  Noncomminuted
  ■ Transverse (Central)
  ■ Polar (Apical or Basal)
  Comminuted
  ■ Stellate
  ■ Transverse
  ■ Polar
  ■ Highly comminuted

KNEE DISLOCATIONS

Descriptive Classification (Figure 3.16)
The position of the tibia relative to the femur defines the direction of dislocation.

Anterior: Forceful knee hyperextension beyond −30 degrees; most common. Associated with posterior (and possibly anterior) cruciate ligament tear, with increasing incidence of popliteal artery disruption with increasing degree of hyperextension.

Posterior: Posteriorly directed force against proximal tibia of flexed knee; "dashboard" injury. Accompanied by anterior and posterior ligament disruption and popliteal artery compromise with increasing proximal tibia displacement.

Lateral: Valgus force. Medial supporting structures disrupted, often with tears of both cruciate ligaments.

Medial: Varus force. Lateral and posterolateral structures disrupted.

Rotational: Varus/valgus with rotatory component. Usually results in buttonholing of the femoral condyle through the articular capsule.

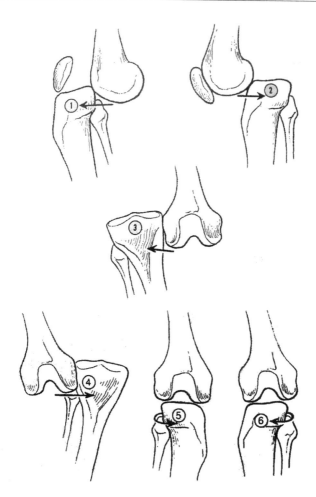

FIGURE 3.16. Classification of knee dislocations.

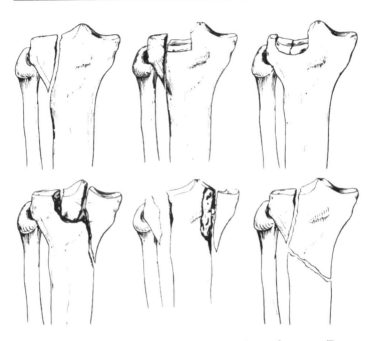

FIGURE 3.17. Schatzker classification of tibial plateau fractures. (Reproduced with permission from Lippincott Williams & Wilkins. Schatzker J. McBroom R. Bruce D. The tibial plateau fracture: the Toronto experience 1968–1975. *Clin Orthop* 1979;138:94–104.)

Tibial Plateau Fractures

Schatzker Classification (Figure 3.17)

Type I: Lateral plateau, split fracture.
Type II: Lateral plateau, split depression fracture.
Type III: Lateral plateau, depression fracture.
Type IV: Medial plateau fracture.
Type V: Bicondylar plateau fracture.
Type VI: Plateau   fracture   with   metaphyseal-diaphyseal dissociation.

Tibial/Fibular Shaft

Descriptive Classification

■ Open versus closed
■ Anatomic location: proximal, middle, or distal third
■ Fragment number and position: comminution, butterfly fragments
■ Configuration: transverse, spiral, oblique
■ Angulation: varus/valgus, anterior/posterior
■ Shortening
■ Displacement: percentage of cortical contact
■ Rotation
■ Associated injuries

Gustilo and Anderson Classification of All Open Fractures

Type I

■ Wound less than 1 cm long
■ Moderately clean puncture, where spike of bone has pierced the skin
■ Little soft tissue damage
■ No crushing
■ Fracture usually simple transverse or oblique with little comminution

Type II

■ Laceration more than 1 cm long
■ No extensive soft tissue damage, flap or contusion
■ Slight to moderate crushing injury
■ Moderate comminution
■ Moderate contamination

Type III

■ Extensive damage to soft tissues
■ High degree of contamination
■ Fracture caused by high velocity trauma

IIIA: Adequate soft tissue cover
IIIB: Inadequate soft tissue cover, a local or free flap is required
IIIC: Any fracture with an arterial injury which requires repair

Pilon Fracture

Ruedi-Allgower Classification (Figure 3.18)

Type 1: No significant articular incongruity; cleavage fractures without displacement of bony fragments.

Type 2: Significant articular incongruity with minimal impaction or comminution.

Type 3: Significant articular comminution with metaphyseal impaction.

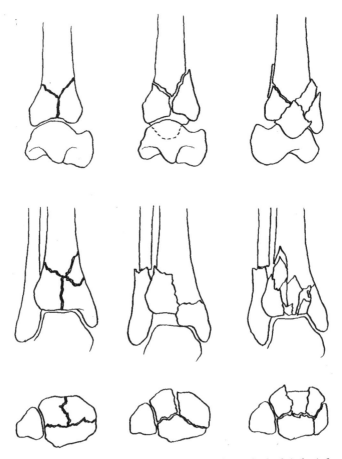

FIGURE 3.18. Ruedi-Allgower classification of distal tibial (pilon) fractures. (Adapted from Muller ME, Narzarian S, Koch P, et al. *Manual of internal fixation*, 2nd ed. New York, Springer-Verlag, 1979:279. Reproduced with kind permission of Springer Science, Business & Media.)

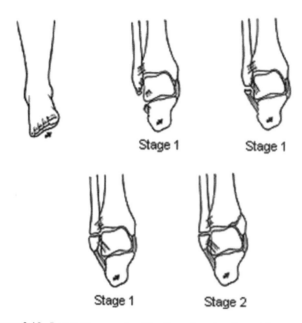

FIGURE 3.19. Lauge-Hansen classification of supination-adduction of the ankle.

ANKLE

Lauge-Hansen Classification (Figure 3.19)
Four patterns, based on "pure" injury sequences, each subdivided into stages of increasing severity.

■ Based on cadaveric studies.
■ Patterns may not always reflect clinical reality.
■ System takes into account the position of the foot at the time of injury and the direction of the deforming force.

Supination-Adduction (SA)
Stage I: Transverse avulsion-type fracture of the fibula distal to the level of the joint or a rupture of the lateral collateral ligaments.
Stage II: Vertical fracture of medial malleolus.

Supination-External Rotation (SER) (Figure 3.20)

Stage I: Disruption of the anterior tibiofibular ligament with or without an associated avulsion fracture at its tibial or fibular attachment.

Stage II: Spiral fracture of the distal fibula, which runs from anteroinferior to posterosuperior.

Stage III: Disruption of the posterior tibiofibular ligament or a fracture of the posterior malleolus.

Stage IV: Transverse avulsion-type fracture of the medial malleolus or a rupture of the deltoid ligament.

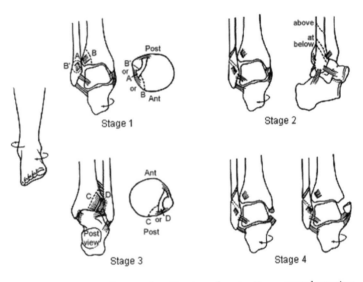

FIGURE 3.20. Lauge-Hansen classification of supination-external rotation of the ankle.

Pronation-Abduction (PA) (Figure 3.21)

Stage I: Transverse fracture of the medial malleolus or a rupture of the deltoid ligament.

Stage II: Rupture of the syndesmotic ligaments or an avulsion fracture at their insertions.

Stage III: Transverse or short oblique fracture of the distal fibula at or above the level of the syndesmosis.

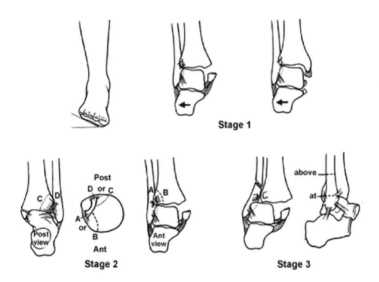

FIGURE 3.21. Lauge-Hansen classification of pronation-abduction of the ankle.

Pronation-External Rotation (PER) (Figure 3.22)

Stage I: Transverse fracture of the medial malleolus or a rupture of the deltoid ligament.

Stage II: Disruption of the anterior tibiofibular ligament with or without an avulsion fracture at its insertion sites.

Stage III: Short oblique fracture of the distal fibula at or above the level of the syndesmosis.

Stage IV: Rupture of the posterior tibiofibular ligament or an avulsion fracture of the posterolateral tibia.

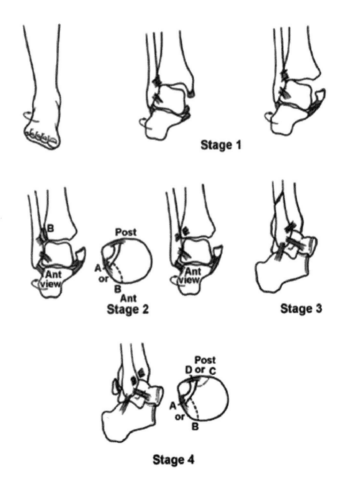

FIGURE 3.22. Lauge-Hansen classification of pronation-external rotation of the ankle.

Pronation – Dorsiflexion (PDA) (Figure 3.23)

Stage I: Fracture of medial malleolus.
Stage II: Fracture of anterior margin of tibia.
Stage III: Supramalleolar fracture of fibula.
Stage IV: Transverse fracture of posterior tibial surface.

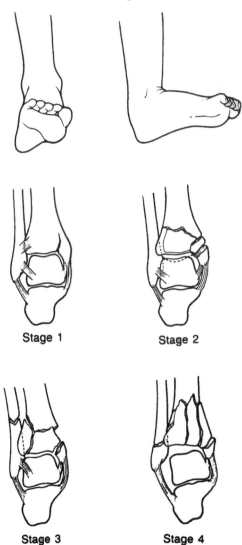

FIGURE 3.23. Lauge-Hansen classification of pronation-dorsiflextion of the ankle.

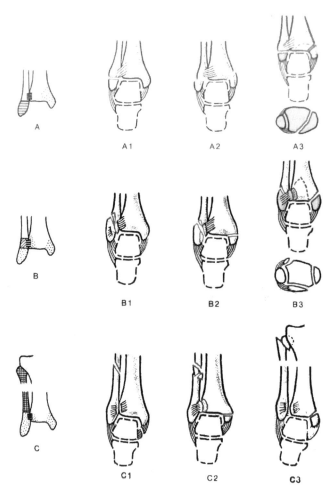

FIGURE 3.24. Danis-Weber classification. (From Muller ME, Nazarian S, Koch P. *The AO Classification of Fractures*. Berlin, Springer–Verlag, 1987. Reproduced with kind permission of Springer Science, Business & Media.)

Danis-Weber Classification (Figure 3.24)

Type A: Fibula fracture below the syndesmosis
      Type A1: Isolated
      Type A2: With fracture of medial malleolus
      Type A3: With posteromedial fracture
Type B: Fibula fracture at the level of syndesmosis
      Type B1: Isolated

Type B2: With medial lesion (malleolus or ligament)
Type B3: With medial lesion and fracture of posterolateral tibia
Type C: Fibula fracture above syndesmosis
Type C1: Diaphyseal fracture of the fibula, simple
Type C2: Diaphyseal fracture of the fibula, complex
Type C3: Proximal fracture of fibula

FOOT

Anatomic Classification of Talus Fractures
■ Lateral process fractures
■ Posterior process fractures
■ Talar head fractures
■ Talar body fractures
■ Talar neck fractures

Hawkins Classification of Talar Neck Fractures (Figure 3.25)
Group I: Nondisplaced
Group II: Associated subtalar subluxation or dislocation

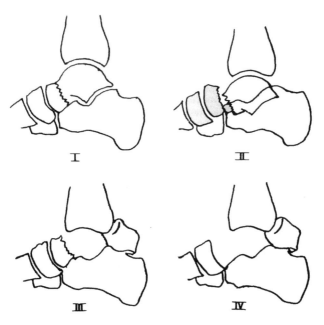

FIGURE 3.25. Hawkins classification of talar neck fractures.

Group III: Associated subtalar and ankle dislocation
Group IV: (Canale and Kelley) Type III with associated talonavicular subluxation or dislocation

Calcaneal Fractures

Classification Of Extraarticular Fractures

■ Anterior process fractures: Due to strong plantar flexion and inversion, which tightens the bifurcate and interosseous ligaments and leads t an avulsion fracture; alternatively, may occur with forefoot abduction with calcaneocuboid compression. Often confused with lateral ankle sprain; seen on lateral or lateral oblique views.

■ Tuberosity fractures: Due to avulsion by the Achilles tendon, especially in diabetics or osteoporotic women, or, rarely, may result from direct trauma; seen on lateral radiographs.

■ Medial process fractures: Vertical shear fracture due to loading of the heel in valgus; seen on axial radiograph.

■ Sustentacular fractures: Occur with heel loading accompanied by severe foot inversion. Often confused with medial ankle sprain; seen on axial radiograph.

■ Body fractures not involving the subtalar articulation: Due to axial loading. Significant comminution, widening, and loss of height may occur along with a reduction in the Bohler angle without posterior facet involvement.

Essex-Lopresti Classification of Intraarticular Fractures
(Figure 3.26)

I. Fractures not involving subtalar joint
   A. Tuberosity fractures
      Beak type
      Avulsion of medial border
      Vertical
      Horizontal
   B. Calcaneocuboid joint only
      Parrot nose
      Various
II. Fractures involving subtalar joint
   A. Without displacement
   B. With displacement
      i. Tongue type
      ii. Centrolateral depression type
      iii. Sustentaculum tali fracture alone

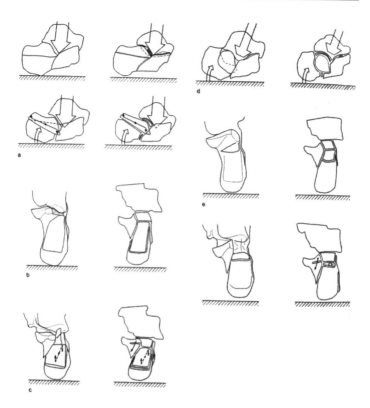

FIGURE 3.26. Essex-Lopresti classification of intraarticular fractures. (From Essex-Lopresti P. Mechanism, reduction techniques and results in fractures of the os calcis. *Br J Surg* 1952;39:395–419.)

    iv. With gross comminution from below, Sever tongue and joint depression type
    v. From behind forward with dislocation of subtalar joint

Souer And Remy Classification
Based on the number of bony fragments determined on Broden, lateral, and Harris axial views:

First degree: Nondisplaced intraarticular fractures
Second degree: Secondary fracture lines resulting in a minimum of three additional pieces, with the posterior main fragment breaking into lateral, middle, and medial fragments
Third degree: Highly comminuted

Sanders Classification (Figure 3.27)

■ Classification based on the number and location of articular fragments as observed by computed tomography and found on the coronal image that shows the widest surface of the inferior facet of the talus.

■ The posterior facet of the calcaneus is divided into three fracture lines (A, B, and C, corresponding to lateral, middle, and medial fracture lines, respectively, on the coronal image).

■ Thus, a total of four potential pieces can result: lateral, central, medial, and sustentaculum tali.

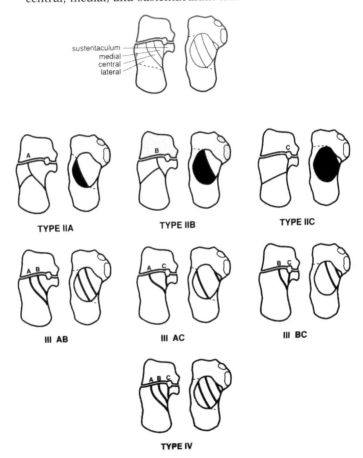

FIGURE 3.27. Sanders Classification. (Reproduced with permission from Lippincott Williams & Wilkins. Sanders R, Fortin P, Di Pasquale T, et al. Operative treatment in 120 displaced intraarticular calcaneal fractures. *Clin Orthop* 1993;290:87–95.)

Type I: All nondisplaced fractures regardless of the number of fracture lines

Type II: Two-part fractures of the posterior facet; subtypes IIA, IIB, IIC based on the location of the primary fracture line

Type III: Three-part fractures in which a centrally depressed fragment exists; subtypes IIIAB, IIIAC, IIIBC

Type IV: Four-part articular fractures; highly comminuted

FRACTURES OF THE MIDFOOT

Midtarsal Joint (Chopart Joint)

Main and Jowett Classification

1. Medial Stress Injury
   - This is an inversion injury with adduction of the midfoot on the hindfoot.
   - Flake fractures of the dorsal margin of the talus or navicular and of the lateral margin of the calcaneus or the cuboid may indicate a sprain.
   - In more severe injuries, the midfoot may be completely dislocated or an isolated talonavicular dislocation may occur. A medial swivel dislocation is one in which the talonavicular joint is dislocated, the subtalar joint is subluxed, and the calcaneocuboid joint is intact.
2. Longitudinal Stress Injury
   - Force is transmitted through the metatarsal heads proximally along the rays, with resultant compression of the midfoot between the metatarsals and the talus with the foot plantar flexed.
   - Longitudinal forces pass between the cuneiforms and fracture the navicular, typically in a vertical pattern.
3. Lateral Stress Injury
   - This s-called "nutcracker fracture" is a characteristic fracture of the cuboid as the forefoot is driven laterally, causing crushing of the cuboid between the calcaneus and the bases of the fourth and fifth metatarsals.
   - This is most commonly an avulsion fracture of the navicular with a comminuted compression fracture of the cuboid.
   - In more severe trauma, the talonavicular joint subluxes laterally and the lateral column of the foot collapses due to comminution of the calcaneocuboid joint.

4. Plantar Stress Injury
   ■ Plantarly directed forces may result in sprains to the mid-tarsal region with avulsion fractures of the dorsal lip of the navicular, talus, or anterior process of the calcaneus.
5. Crush injuries

Navicular Fractures

Eichenholtz And Levin Classification
Type I: Avulsion fractures of tuberosity
Type II: A fracture involving the dorsal lip
Type III: A fracture through the body

Sangeorzan Classification (Figure 3.28)
Type I: Transverse fracture line in the coronal plane, with no angulation of the forefoot
Type II: The major fracture line from dorsolateral to plantar-medial with talonavicular joint disruption and forefoot is displaced laterally

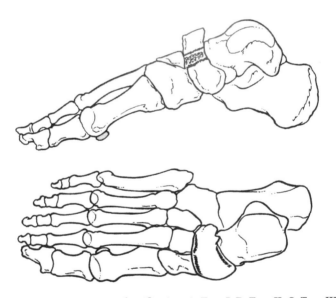

FIGURE 3.28. Sangeorzan classification. A, Type I; B, Type II; C, Type III. (Reproduced with permission and copyright © of The Journal of Bone and Joint Surgery, Inc. Sangeorzan BJ, Benirschke SK, Mosca V, Mayo KA, and Hansen ST Jr: Displaced intra-articular fractures of the tarsal navicular. *J Bone Joint Surg Am* 1989;71A:1504–1510.)

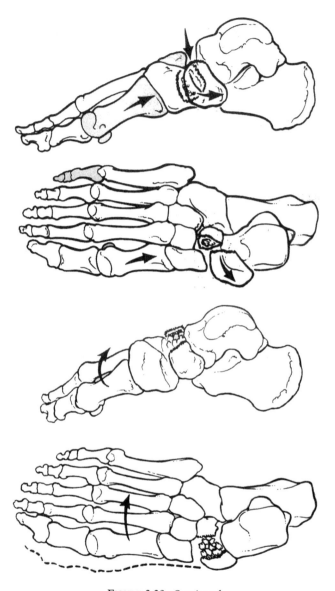

FIGURE 3.28. *Continued*

Type III: Comminuted fracture pattern with naviculo-cuneiform joint disruption; associated fractures may exist (cuboid, anterior calcaneus, calcaneocuboid joints).

Cuboid Fractures

OTA Classification Of Cuboid Fractures

Higher letters and numbers denote more significant injury. Type A: extraarticular, no joint involvement.

Type A: Extraarticular
      Type A1: Extraarticular, avulsion
      Type A2: Extraarticular, coronal
      Type A3: Extraarticular, multifragmentary
Type B: Partial articular, single joint (calcaneocuboid or cubotarsal)
      Type B1: Partial articular, sagittal
      Type B2: Partial articular, horizontal
Type C: Articular, calcaneocuboid and cubotarsal involvement
      Type C1: Articular, multifragmentary
            Type C1.1: Nondisplaced
            Type C1.2: Displaced

Tarsometatarsal (Lisfranc) Joint

Quenu and Kuss Classification (Figure 3.29)
Based on commonly observed patterns of injury.

Type 1: Homolateral. All five metatarsals displaced in the same direction.

Type 2: Isolated. One or two metatarsals displaced form the others.

Type 3: Divergent. Displacement of the metatarsals in both the sagittal and coronal planes.

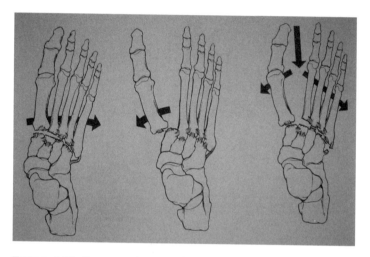

FIGURE 3.29. Quenu and Kuss classification. (From Heckman JD, Bucholz RW, (Eds). Rockwood, Green, and Wilkins' Fractures in Adults. Philadelphia: 2001.)

Myerson Classification (Figure 3.30)
A. Total incongruity
   Lateral
   Dorsoplantar
B. Partial incongruity
   Medial
   Lateral

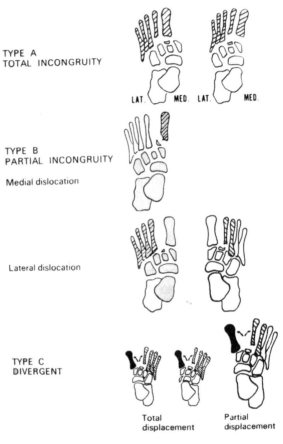

FIGURE 3.30. Myerson classification of Lisfranc fracture-dislocation. (From Myerson MS, Fisher RT, Burgess AR, et al. Fracture-dislocations of the tarsometatarsal joints: end results correlated with pathology and treatment. Copyright © 1986 by the American Orthopaedic Foot and Ankle Society (AOFAS), originally published in Foot and Ankle International, April 1986, Volume 6, Number 5, page 228 and reproduced here with permission.)

C. Divergent
    Partial
    Total

Fractures of the Base of the Fifth Metatarsal

Dameron Classification (Figures 3.31)
Zone 1: Avulsion fractures
Zone 2: Fractures at the metaphyseal-diaphyseal junction (Jone's fracture)
Zone 3: Stress fractures of the proximal 1.5 cm of the shaft of the fifth metatarsal

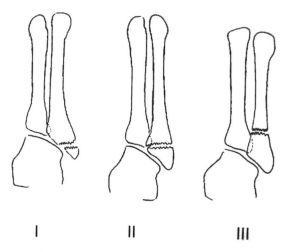

I   II   III

FIGURE 3.31. Dameron & Lawrence & Boote classification.

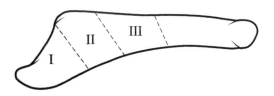

FIGURE 3.32. Dameron classification. (Dameron TB. Fractures of the proximal fifth metatarsal: selecting the best treatment option. ©1995 American Academy of Orthopaedic Surgeons. Reprinted from The Journal of the American Academy of Orthopaedic Surgeons, Volume 3 (2), pp. 110–114 with permission.)

First Metatarsophalangeal Joint

Bowers and Martin Classification

Grade I: Strain at the proximal attachment of the volar plate from the first metatarsal head

Grade II: Avulsion of the volar plate from the metatarsal head

Grade III: Impaction injury to the dorsal surface of the metatarsal head with or without an avulsion or chip fracture

Dislocation of the First Metatarsophalangeal Joint

Jahss Classification

Based on integrity of the sesamoid complex:

Type I: Volar plate is avulsed off the first metatarsal head; proximal phalanx displaced dorsally; intersesamoid ligament remains intact and lies over the dorsum of the metatarsal head

Type II

Type IIA: Intersesamoid ligament is ruptured

Type IIB: Longitudinal fracture of either sesamoid is seen

Chapter 4
Fractures in Children

GENERAL

Salter-Harris Classification (Figure 4.1)

Type I: Transphyseal fracture involving the hypertophic and calcified zones; prognosis is usually excellent, although complete or partial growth arrest may occur in displaced fractures.

Type II: Transphyseal fracture that exits the metaphysis; the metaphyseal fragment is known as the Thurston-Holland fragment; the periosteal hinge is intact on the side with the metaphyseal fragment; prognosis is excellent, although complete or partial growth arrest may occur in displaced fractures.

Type III: Transphyseal fracture that exits the epiphysis, causing intraarticular disruption; anatomic reduction and fixation without violating the physis are essential; prognosis is guarded because partial growth arrest and resultant angular deformity are common problems.

Type IV: Fracture that traverses the epiphysis and the physis, exiting the metaphysis; anatomic reduction and fixation without violating the physis are essential; prognosis is guarded, because partial growth arrest and resultant angular deformity are common.

Type V: Crush injury to the physis; diagnosis is generally made retrospectively; prognosis is poor because growth arrest and partial physeal closure commonly result.

Type VI: (Rang) Bruise or contusion to periphery of the epiphyseal plate. It can cause scaring, tethering and arrest of the periphery of the epiphyseal plate, producing angular deformity.

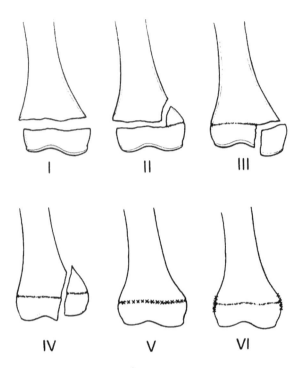

FIGURE 4.1. Salter-Harris classification.

SUPRACONDYLAR HUMERUS FRACTURES

Classification of Extension Type

Gartland Classification
Based on degree of displacement:

Type I: Nondisplaced
Type II: Displaced with intact posterior cortex; may be slightly angulated or rotated
Type III: Complete displacement; Posteromedial or postero-lateral

Wilkins Modification of Gartland's Classification
Type 1: Undisplaced

Type 2
> Type 2A: Intact posterior cortex and angulation only
> Type 2B: Intact posterior cortex, angulation and rotation

Type 3
> Type 3A: Completely displaced, no cortical contact, posteromedial
> Type 3B: Completely displaced, no cortical contact, posterolateral

LATERAL CONDYLAR PHYSEAL FRACTURES

Milch Classification (Figure 4.2)

Type I: Fracture line courses lateral to the trochlea and into the capitelotrochlear groove, representing a Salter-Harris type IV fracture. The elbow is stable because the trochlea is intact.

Type II: Fracture line extends into the apex of the trochlea, representing a Salter-Harris type II fracture. The elbow is unstable because the trochlea is disrupted.

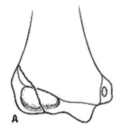

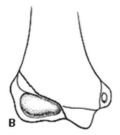

FIGURE 4.2. Milch Classification. (From Milch H. Fractures and fracture dislocations of the humeral condyles. *J Trauma* 1964;4:592–604.)

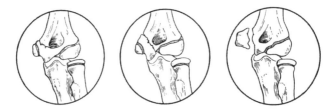

FIGURE 4.3. Kilfoyle classification. (Reproduced with permission from Lippincott Williams & Wilkins. Kilfoyle RM. Fractures of the medial condyle and epicondyle of the elbow in children. *Clin Orthop* 41: 43–50.)

MEDIAL CONDYLAR PHYSEAL FRACTURES

Kilfoyle Classification (Figure 4.3)

Type I: Impacted or greenstick fracture

Type II: A fracture through the humeral condyle into the joint with little or no displacement

Type III: An epiphyseal fracture that is intraarticular and involves the medial condyle with the fragment displaced and rotated

TRANSPHYSEAL FRACTURES

Delee Classification

Based on ossification of the lateral condyle:

Group A: Infant, before appearance of lateral condylar ossification centre (birth to 7 months of age); diagnosis easily missed; Salter-Harris type I.

Group B: Lateral condyle ossified (7 months to 3 years); Salter-Harris type I or II (fleck of metaphysis).

Group C: Large metaphyseal fragment, usually exiting laterally (ages 3 to 7 years).

T-CONDYLAR FRACTURES

Wilkins and Beaty Classification

Type I: Nondisplaced or minimally displaced

Type II: Displaced, with no metaphyseal comminution

Type III: Displaced, with metaphyseal comminution

RADIAL HEAD AND NECK FRACTURES

Wilkins Classification (Figure 4.4)

Type A: Salter-Harris Type I or II physeal injury

Type B: Salter-Harris Type III or IV intraarticular injury

Type C: Fracture line completely within metaphysic

Type D: Fractures occurring when a dislocated elbow is being reduced

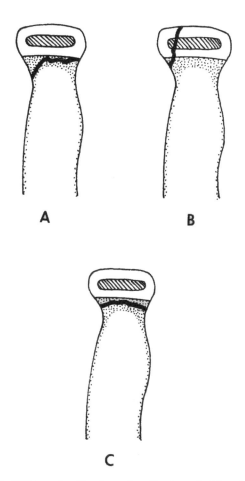

FIGURE 4.4. Wilkins classification of pediatric radial head and neck fractures.

Type E: Fracture occurring with elbow dislocation
- Fracture associated with elbow dislocation
  Reduction injury
  Dislocation injury

Letts Classification of Monteggia Fracture Dislocation
(Figure 4.5)
Dislocation of the radial head with fracture of ulna

1. Anterior bend
2. Anterior greenstick
3. Anterior complete
4. Posterior
5. Lateral

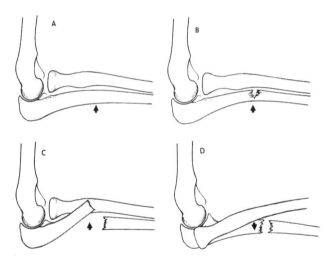

FIGURE 4.5. Letts classification of Monteggia fracture dislocation.

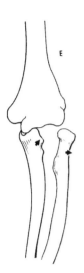

FIGURE 4.5. *Continued*

PEDIATRIC FOREARM

Descriptive Classification
Location: Proximal, middle, or distal third
Type: Plastic deformation, incomplete ("greenstick"), compression ("torus" or "buckle"), or complete displacement angulation
Associated physeal injuries: Salter-Harris Types I to V

SCAPHOID

Classification
Type A: Fractures of the distal pole
        Type A1: Extraarticular distal pole fractures
        Type A2: Intraarticular distal pole fractures
Type B: Fractures of the middle third
Type C: Fractures of the proximal pole

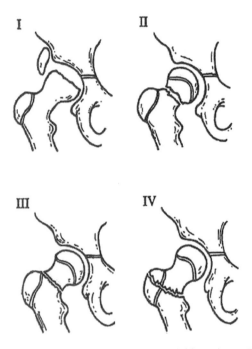

FIGURE 4.6. Classification of hip fractures in children. (From Rockwood CA Jr, Wilkins KE, Beaty JH, eds. *Rockwood and Green's fractures in children*, 4th ed. Vol. 3. Philadelphia, Lippincott-Raven, 1996:1151.)

PEDIATRIC HIP FRACTURES (Figure 4.6)

Delbet Classification of Pediatric Hip Fractures

Type I: Transepiphyseal fracture
Type II: Transcervical fracture
Type III: Cervicotrochanteric fracture
Type IV: Intertrochanteric fracture

TIBIAL SPINE (INTERCONDYLAR EMINENCE) FRACTURES

Meyers and McKeever Classification (Figure 4.7)

Type I: Minimal or no displacement of fragment

Type II: Angular elevation of anterior portion with intact posterior hinge

Type III: Complete displacement with or without rotation

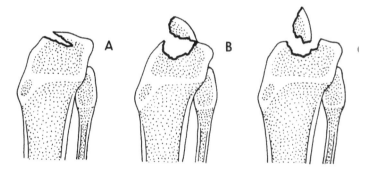

FIGURE 4.7. Meyers and McKeever classification.

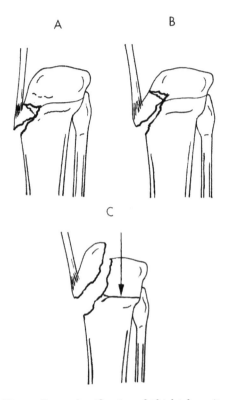

FIGURE 4.8. Watson-Jones classification of tibial tuberosity fractures.

TIBIAL TUBEROSITY FRACTURE

Watson-Jones Classification (Figure 4.8)

Type I: A small fragment, displaced superiorly

Type II: A larger fragment involving the secondary centre of ossification and proximal tibial epiphysis

Type III: A fracture that passes proximally and posteriorly across the epiphyseal plate and proximal articular surface of tibia (Salter-Harris Type III)

CALCANIAL FRACTURES

Schmidt and Weiner Classification of Calcaneal Fractures

Type I: Fracture of the tuberosity of apophyses
　　　Type IA: Fracture of the sustentaculum
　　　Type IB: Fracture of the anterior process
　　　Type IC: Fracture of the anterior inferolateral process
　　　Type ID: Avulsion fracture of the body
Type II: Fracture of the posterior and/or superior parts of the tuberosity
Type III: Fracture of the body not involving the subtalar joint
Type IV: Nondisplaced or minimally displaced fracture through the subtalar joint
Type V: Displaced fracture through the subtalar joint
　　　Type VA: Tongue type
　　　Type VB: Joint depression type
Type VI: Either unclassified or serious soft-tissue injury, bone loss, and loss of the insertions of the Achilles tendon

Chapter 5
Periprosthetic Fractures

PERIPROSTHETIC HIP FRACTURES

Vancouver Classification (Duncan and Masri)

Type A: Involve the trochanteric area (AG involve the greater trochanter, AL involve the lesser trochanter)

Type B: Fractures around the stem or extending slightly distal to it (B1 implant well fixed, B2 implant loose, bone stock adequate, B3 implant loose, bone stock inadequate)

Type C: Fractures distal to the stem that the presence of the femoral component may be ignored

Johansson Classification

Type I: Fracture proximal to prosthetic tip with the stem remaining in the medullary canal

Type II: Fracture extending beyond distal stem with dislodgement of the stem from the distal canal

Type III: Fracture entirely distal to the tip of the prosthesis

Cooke And Newman (Modification Of Bethea) (Figure 5.1)

Type I: Explosion type with comminution around the stem; the prosthesis is always loose, and the fracture is inherently unstable

Type II: Oblique fracture around the stem; fracture pattern is stable, but prosthetic loosening usually is present

Type III: Transverse fracture at the distal tip of the stem; the fracture is unstable, but prosthetic fixation is usually unaffected

Type IV: Fracture entirely distal to prosthesis; fracture is unstable, but prosthetic fixation is usually unaffected

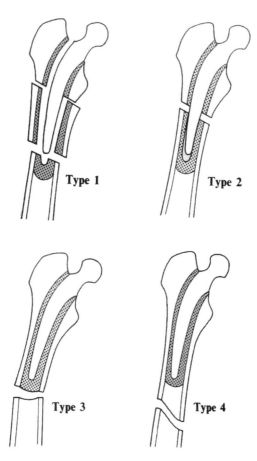

FIGURE 5.1. Cooke and Newman classification of periprosthetic fracture about total hip implants. (Reproduced with permission and copyright © of the British Editorial Society of Bone and Joint Surgery. Cooke PH, Newman JH. Fractures of the femur in relation to cemented hip prostheses. *J Bone Joint Surg Br* 1988;70B:386.)

PERIPROSTHETIC KNEE FRACTURES

FEMORAL FRACTURES

Lewis and Rorabeck Classification
Type I: Undisplaced fractures, prosthesis intact
Type II: Displaced fractures, prosthesis intact
Type III: Displaced or undisplaced fracture, prosthesis loose or failing

Neer Classification, With Modification by Merkel (Figure 5.2)
Type I: Minimally displaced supracondylar fracture
Type II: Displaced supracondylar fracture
Type III: Comminuted supracondylar fracture
Type IV: Fracture at the tip of the prosthetic femoral stem of the diaphysis above the prosthesis
Type V: Any fracture of the tibia

TIBIAL FRACTURES (NEER AND MERKEL TYPE V)

Goldberg Classification
Type I: Fractures not involving cement/implant composite or quadriceps mechanism
Type II: Fractures involving cement/implant composite and/or quadriceps mechanism
Type III
        Type IIIA: Inferior pole fractures with patellar ligament disruption
        Type IIIB: Inferior pole fractures without patellar ligament disruption
Type IV: Fracture-dislocation

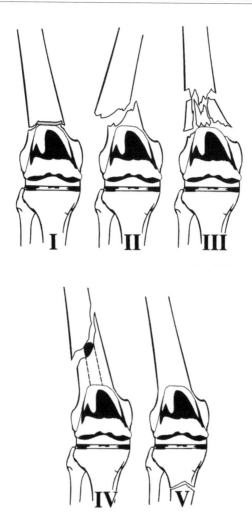

FIGURE 5.2. Periprosthetic fracture of the knee. (From Neer C, Grantham
S, Shelton M. Supracondylar fracture of the adult femur. A study of 110
cases. *J Bone Joint Surg Am* 1967;49A; 591. Reproduced with permission
and copyright © of The Journal of Bone and Joint Surgery, Inc. Merkel
KD, Johnson EW Jr. Supracondylar fracture of the femur after total knee
arthroplasty. *J Bone Joint Surg Am* 1986;68A:29–43.)

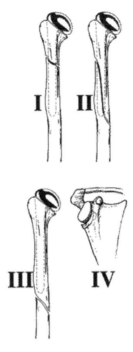

FIGURE 5.3. Periprosthetic fracture of the shoulder. (From Rockwood CA, Green DP, Bucholz RW, Heckman JD. *Rockwood and Green's fractures in adults*, 4th ed. Philadelphia, Lippincott-Raven, 1996:543.)

PERIPROSTHETIC SHOULDER FRACTURES

University of Texas at San Antonio Classification (Figure 5.3)

Type I: Fractures occurring proximal to the tip of the humeral prosthesis

Type II: Fractures occurring in the proximal portion of the humerus with distal extension beyond the tip of the humeral prosthesis

Type III: Fractures occurring entirely distal to the tip of the humeral prosthesis

Type IV: Fractures occurring adjacent to the glenoid prosthesis

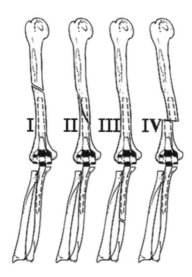

FIGURE 5.4. Periprosthetic elbow fractures. (From Heckman JD, Bucholz RW, eds. *Rockwood, Green, and Wilkins' Fractures in Adults*. Philadelphia, Lippincott Williams & Wilkins, 2001.)

PERIPROSTHETIC ELBOW FRACTURES (Figure 5.4)

Classification

Type I: Fracture of the humerus proximal to the humeral component

Type II: Fracture of the humerus or ulna in any location along the length of the prosthesis

Type III: Fracture of the ulna distal to the ulnar component

Type IV: Fracture of the implant

Index